MY LOCAL HOSPITAL

H

Alan Walker

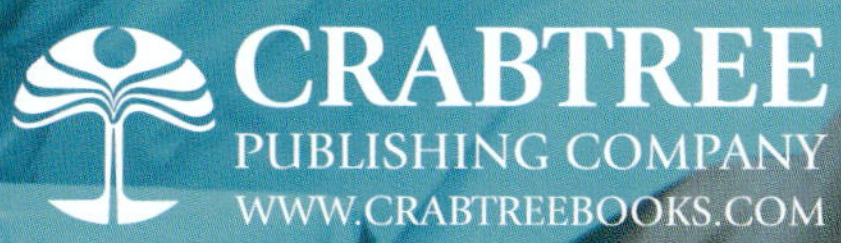

My **local hospital** has lots of rooms!

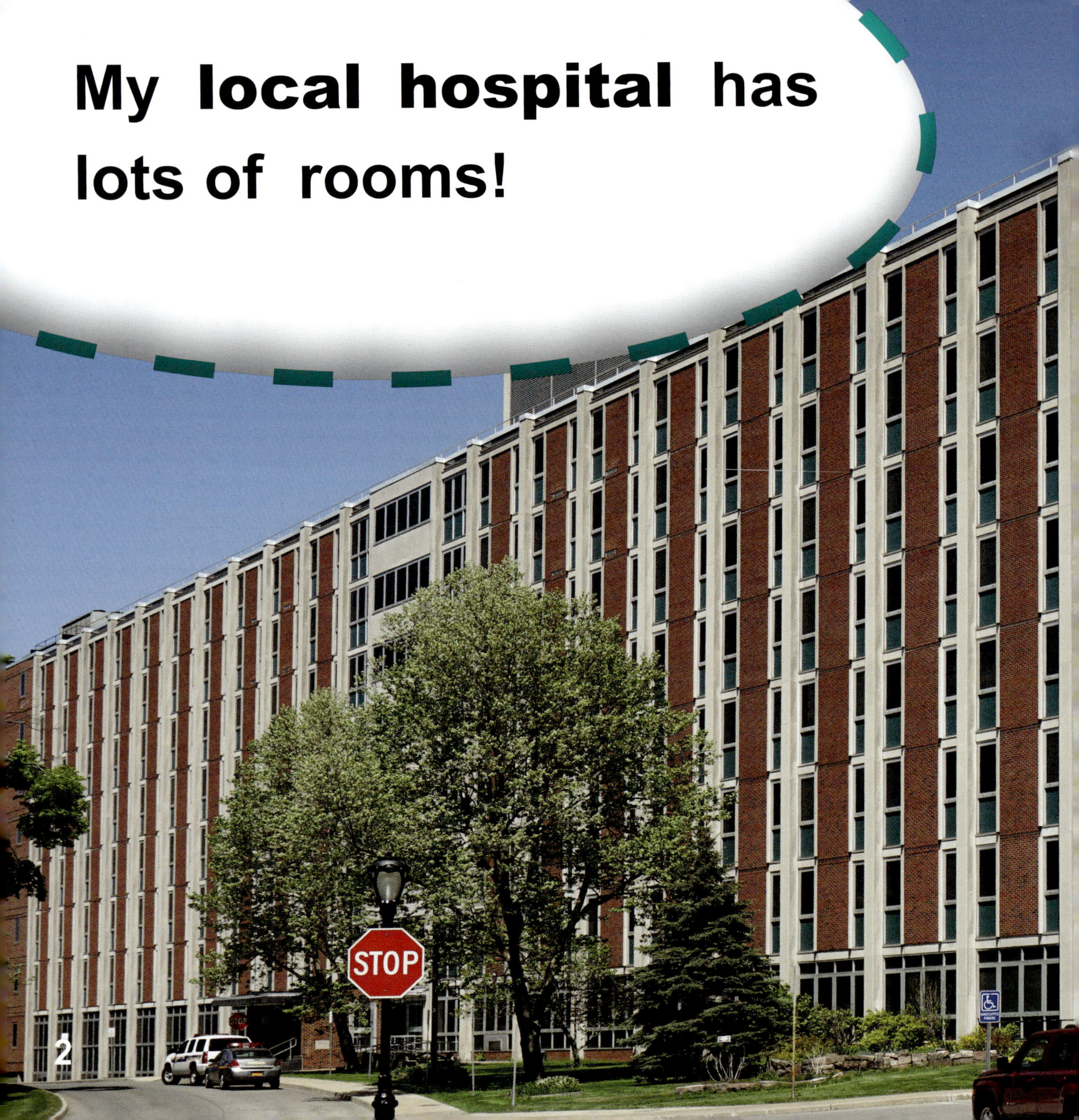

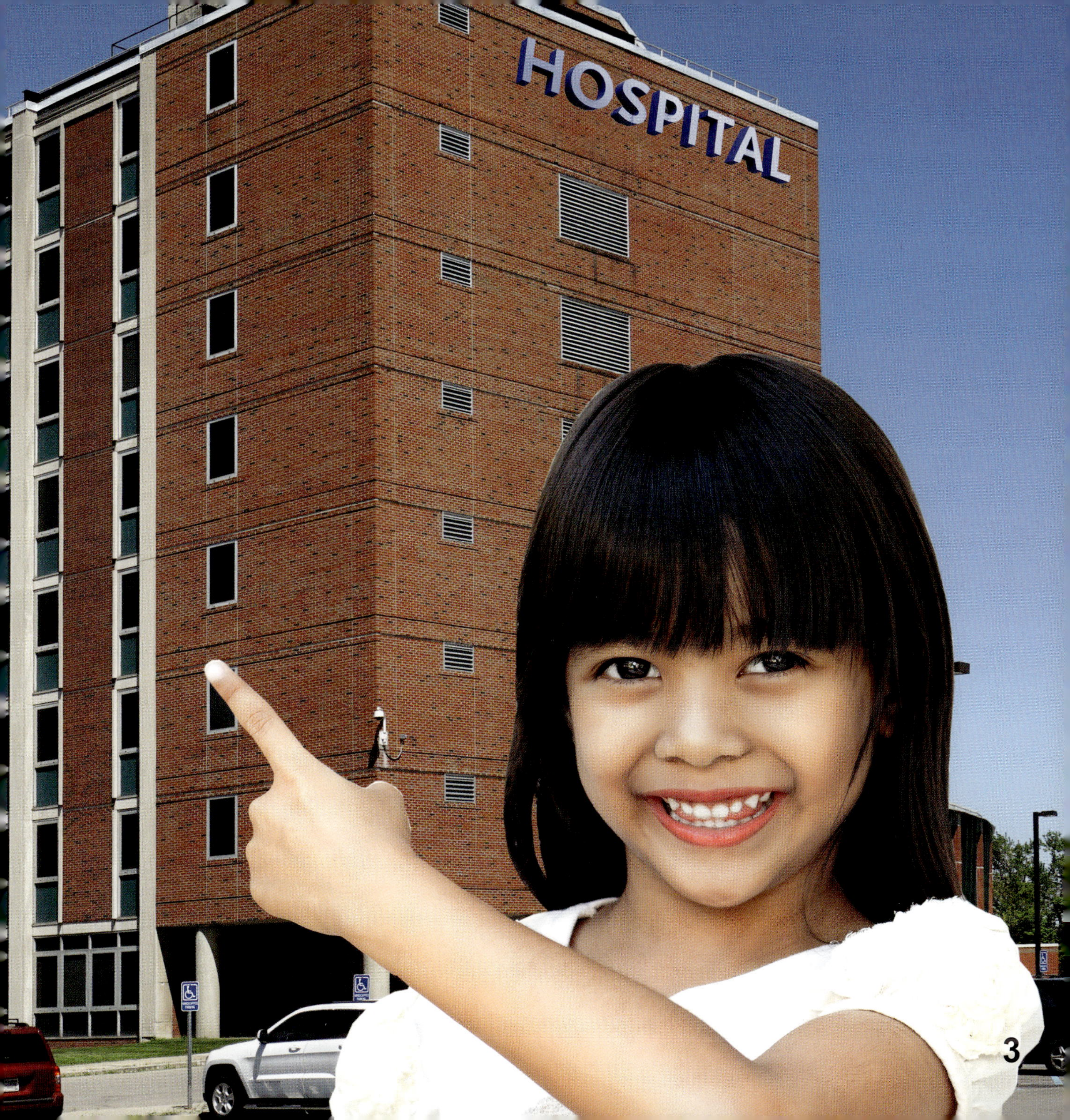
HOSPITAL

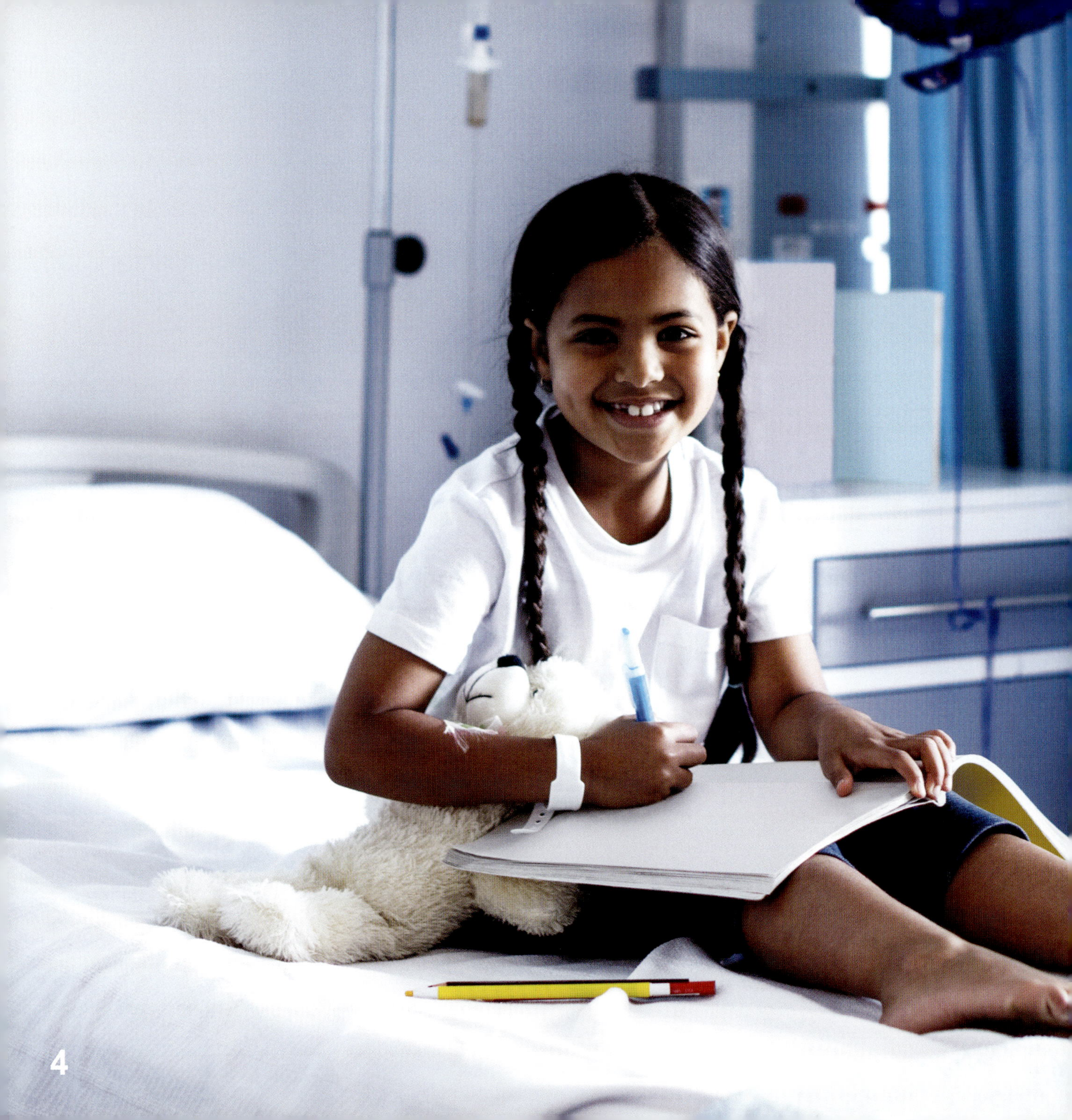

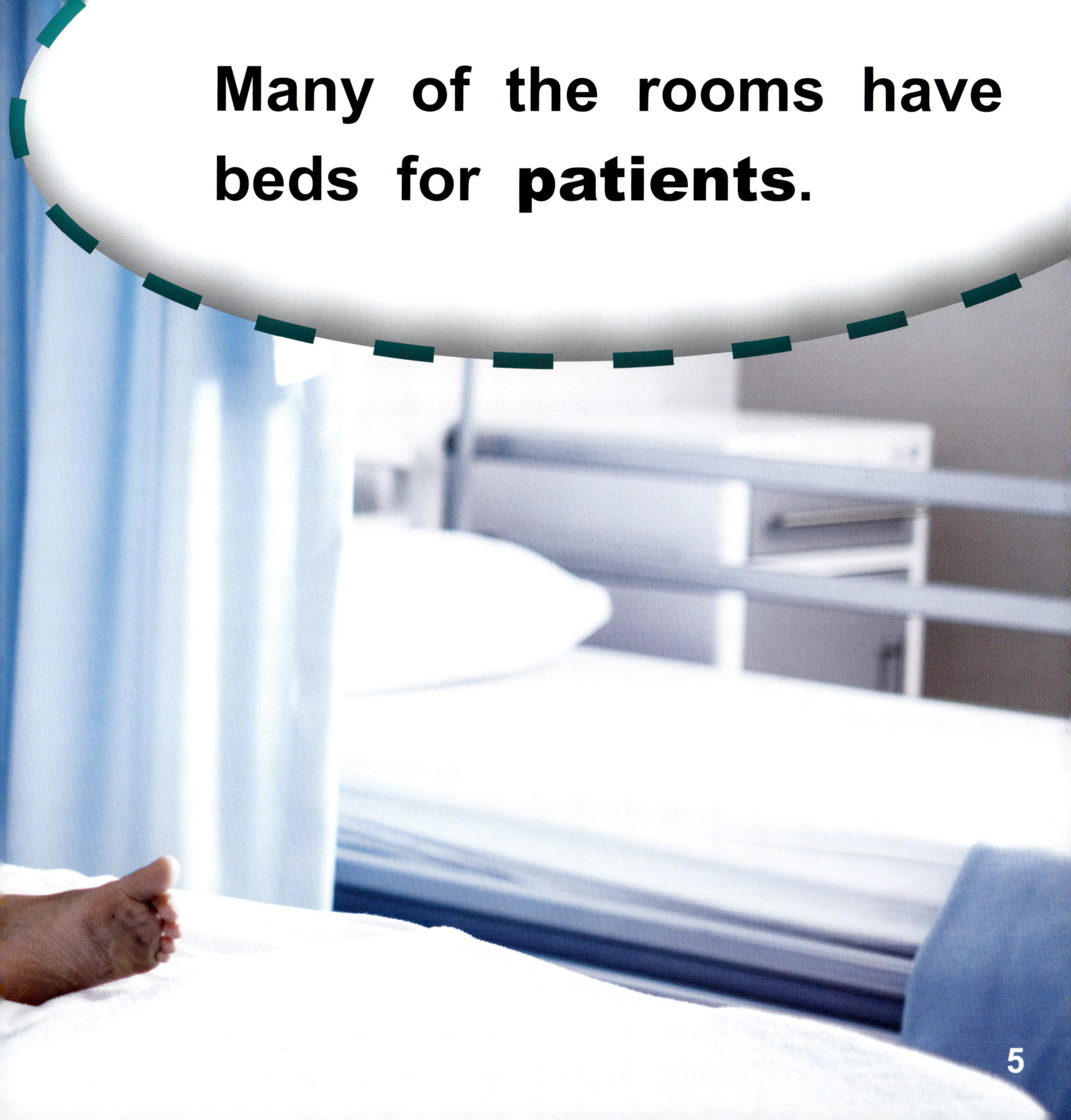

Many of the rooms have beds for **patients**.

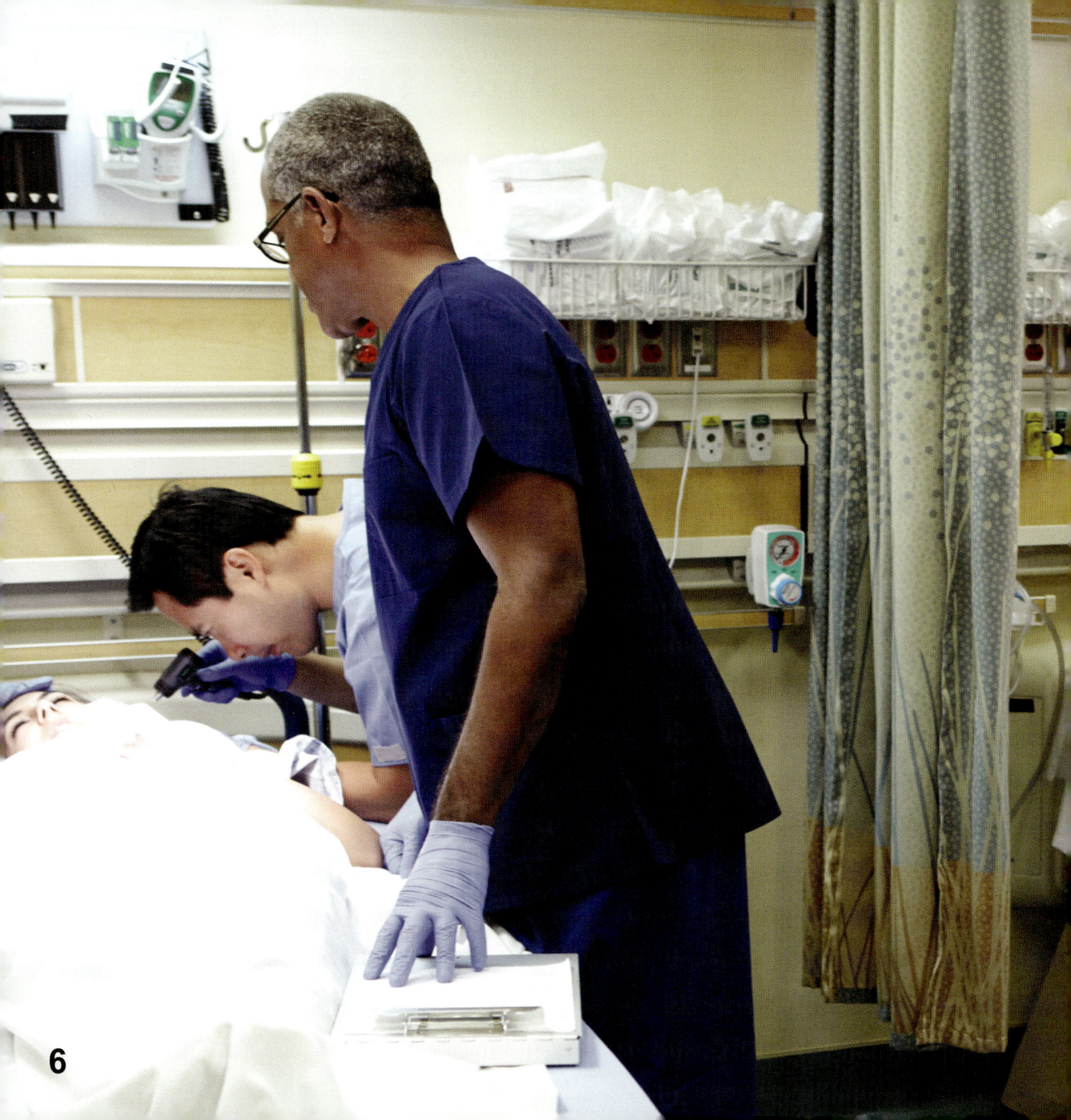

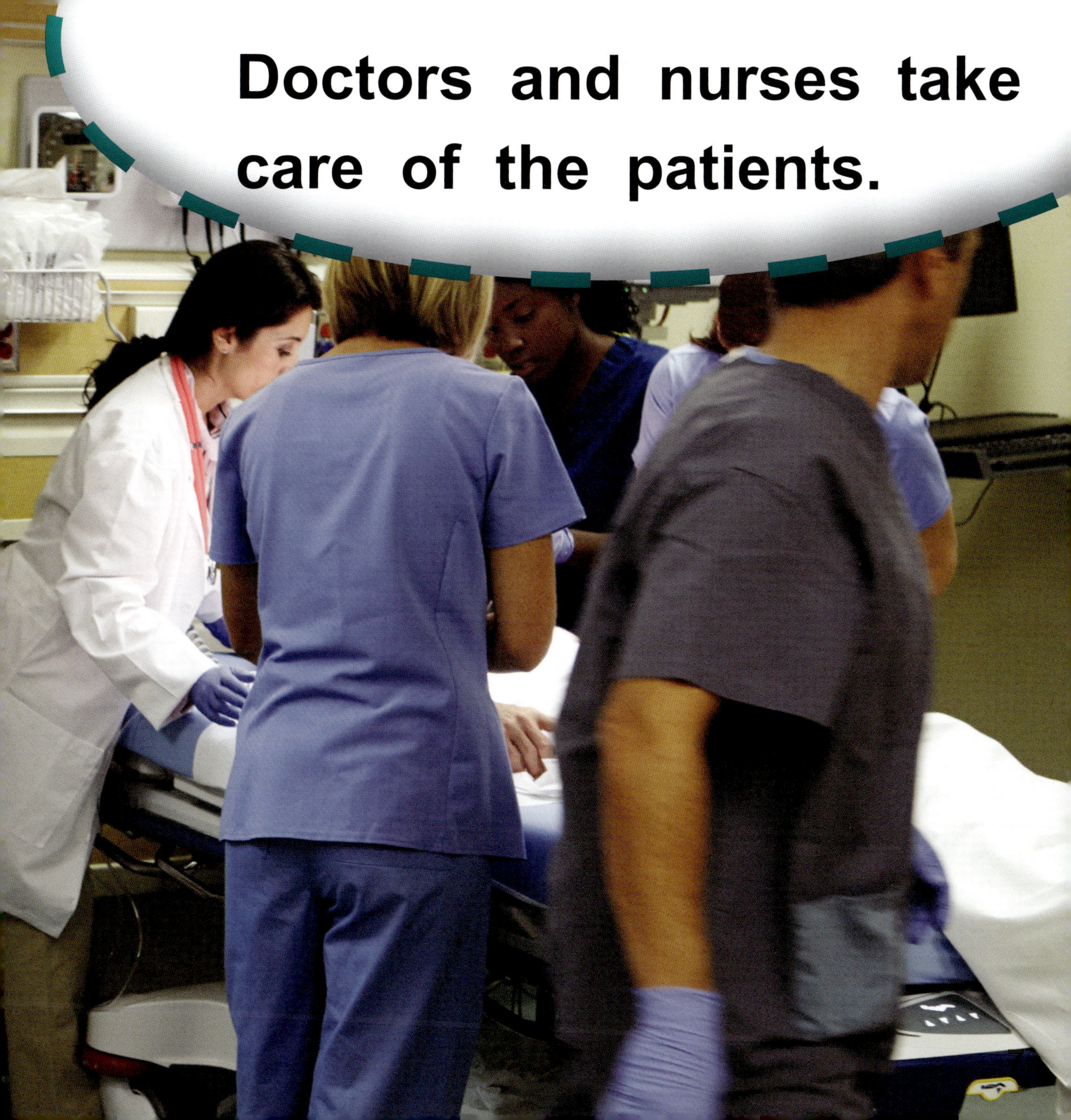

Doctors and nurses take care of the patients.

My local hospital has an **operating room.**

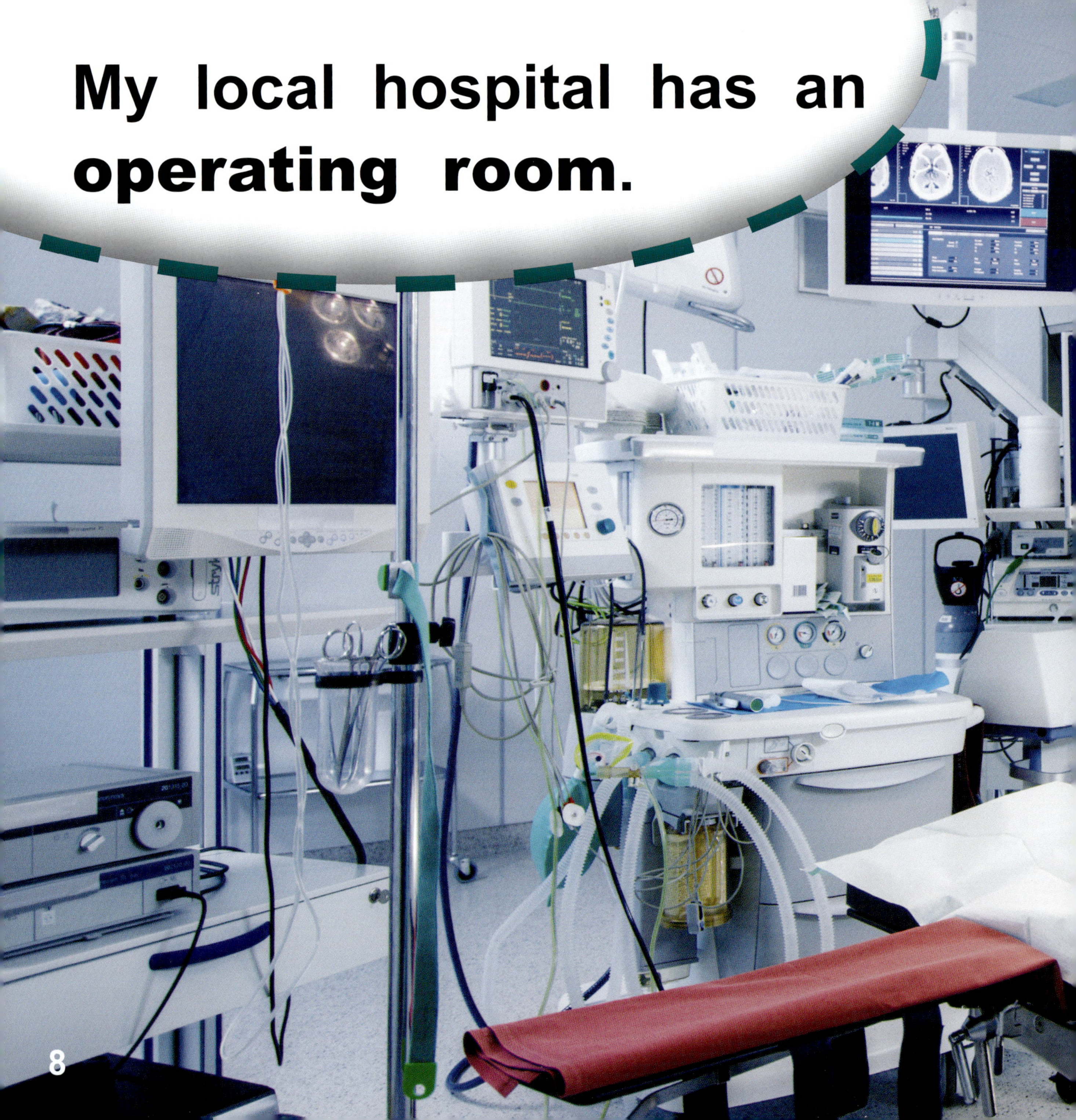

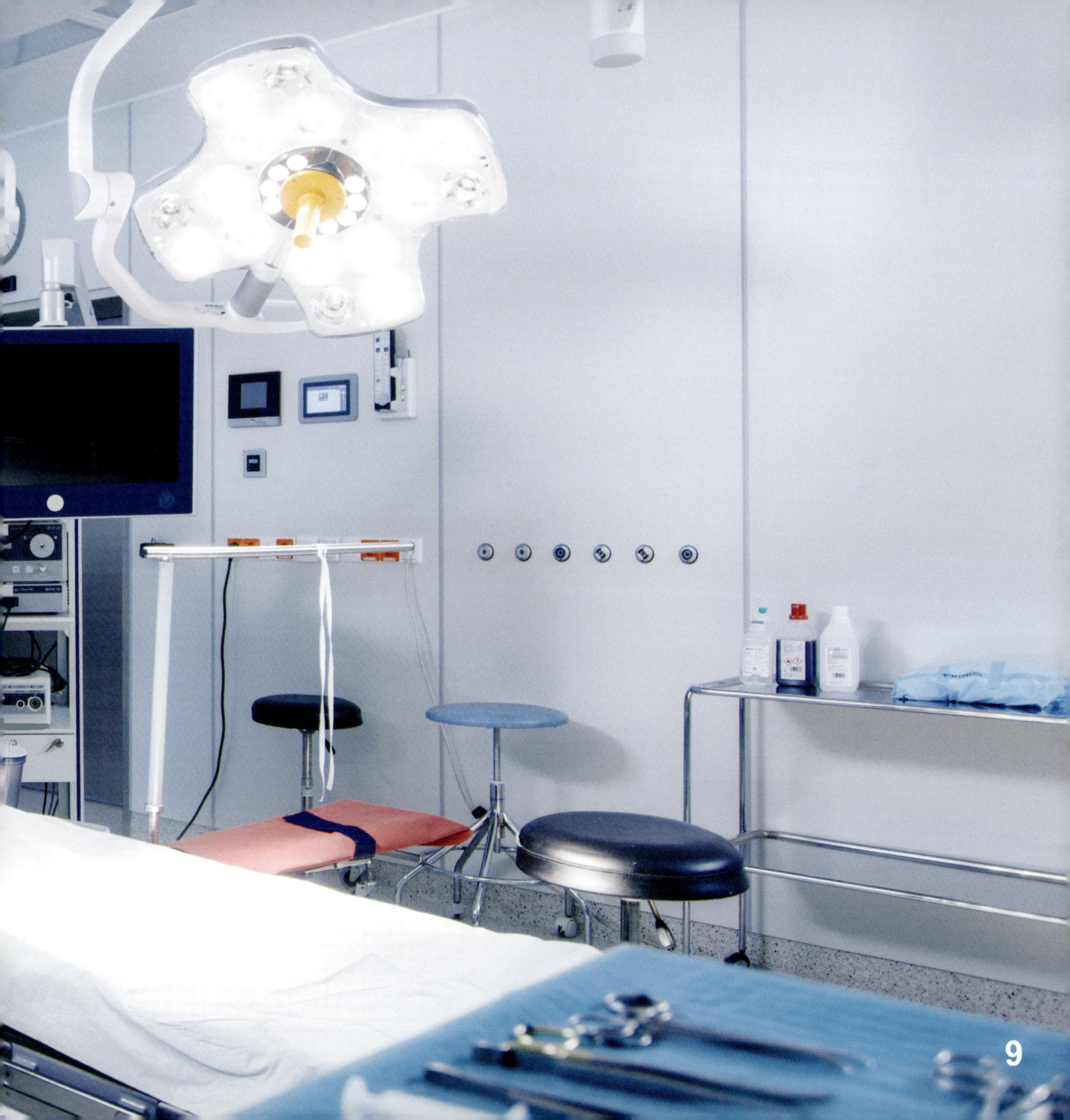

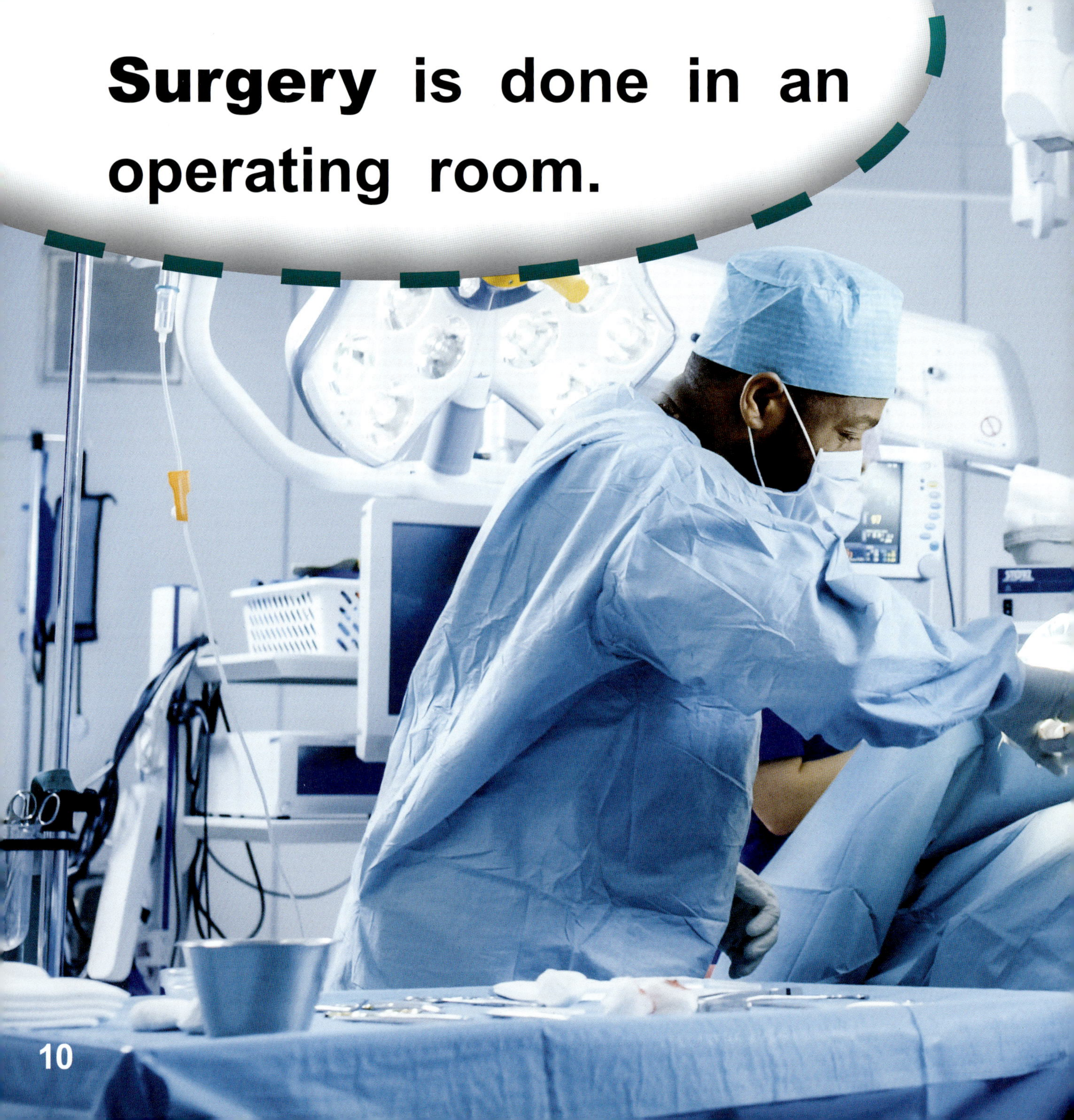

Surgery is done in an operating room.

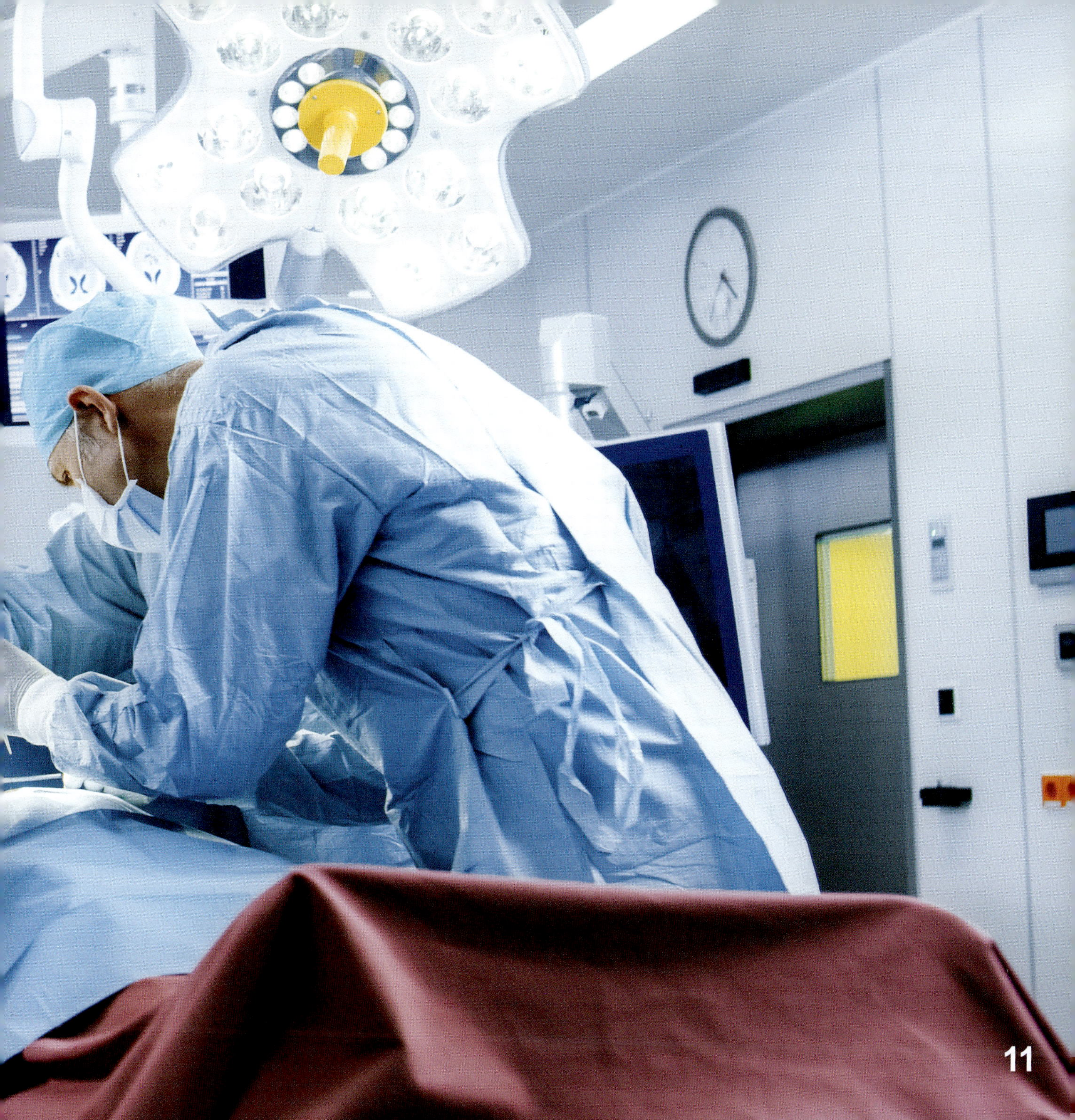

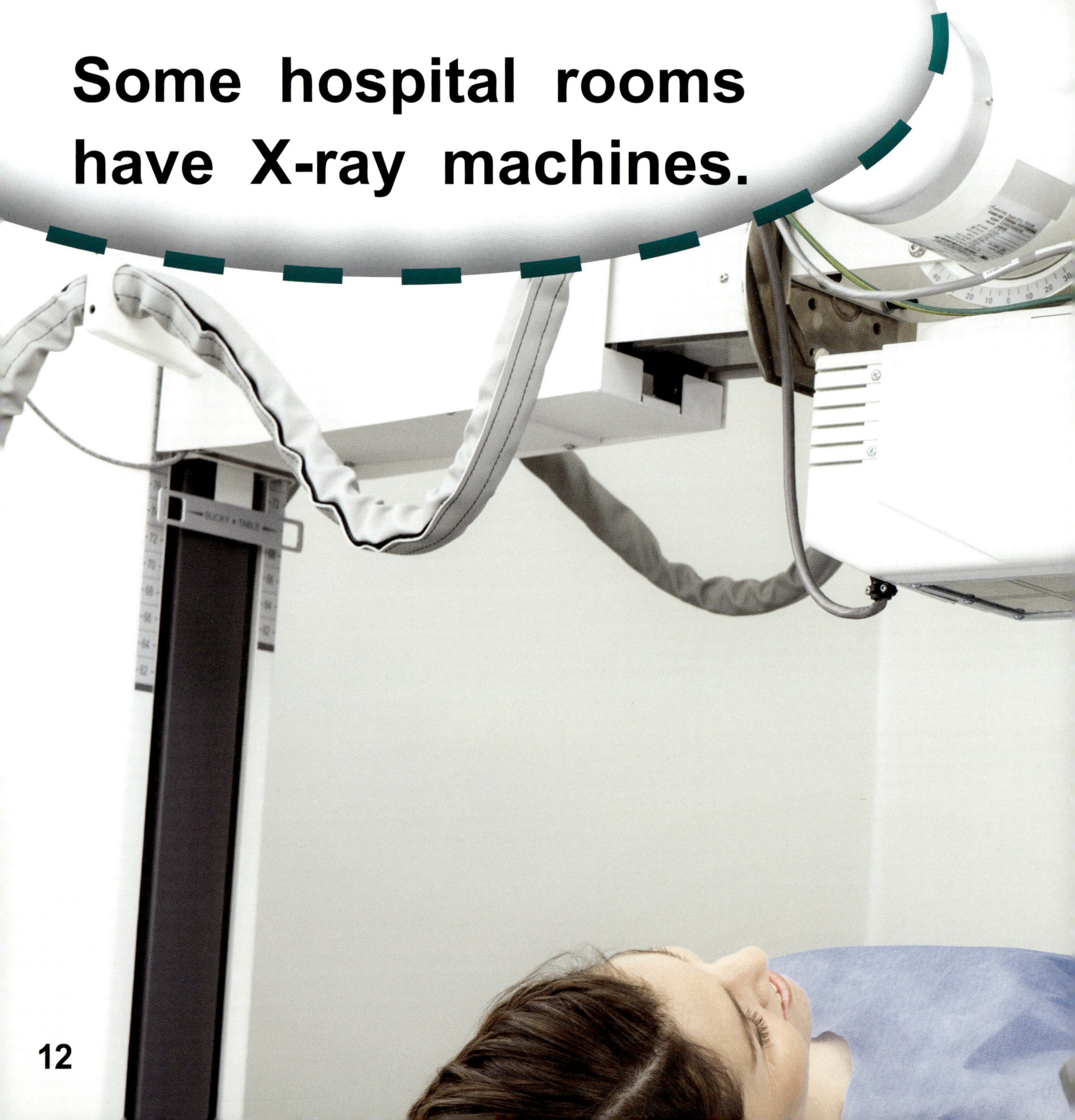

Some hospital rooms have X-ray machines.

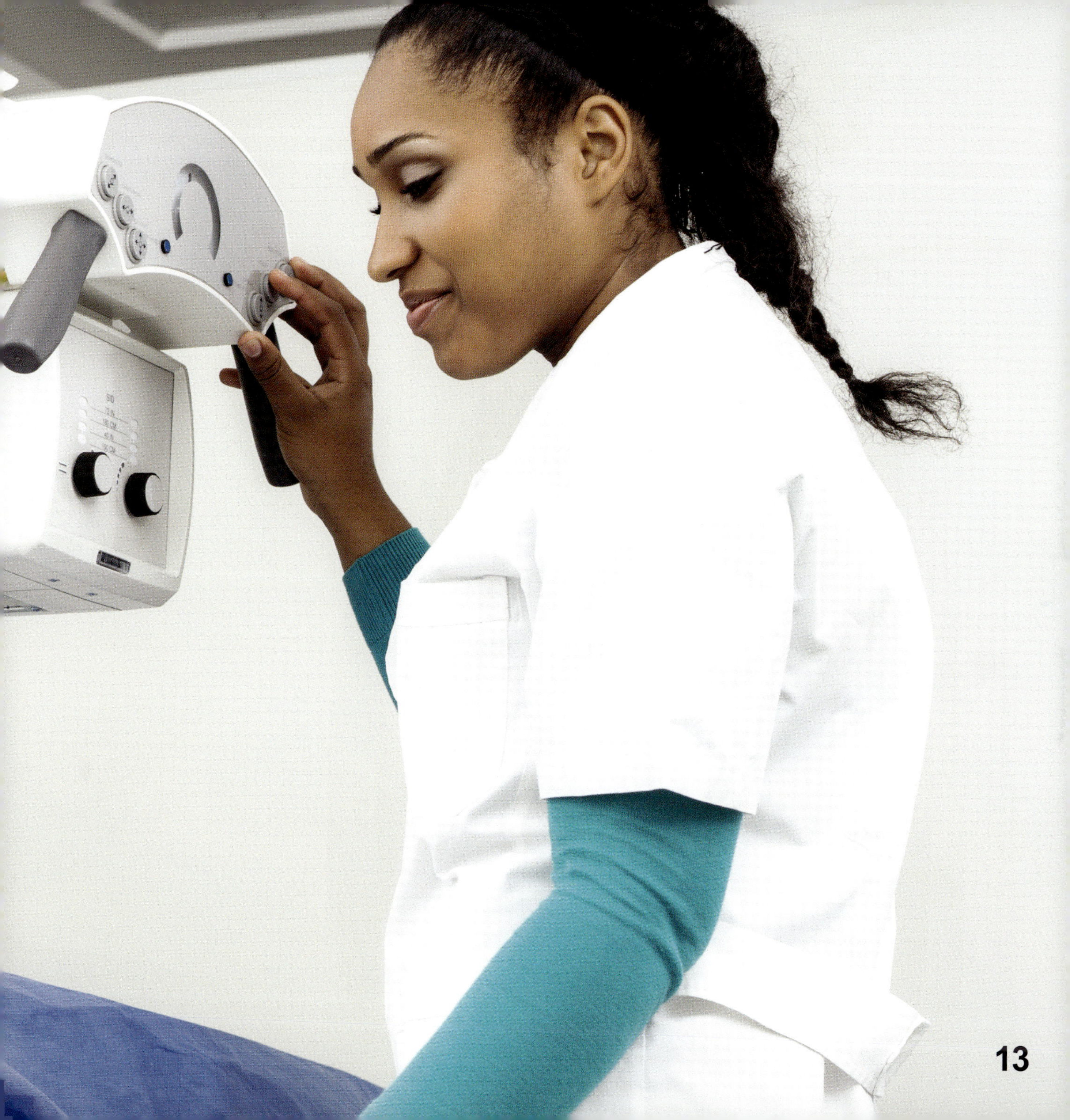

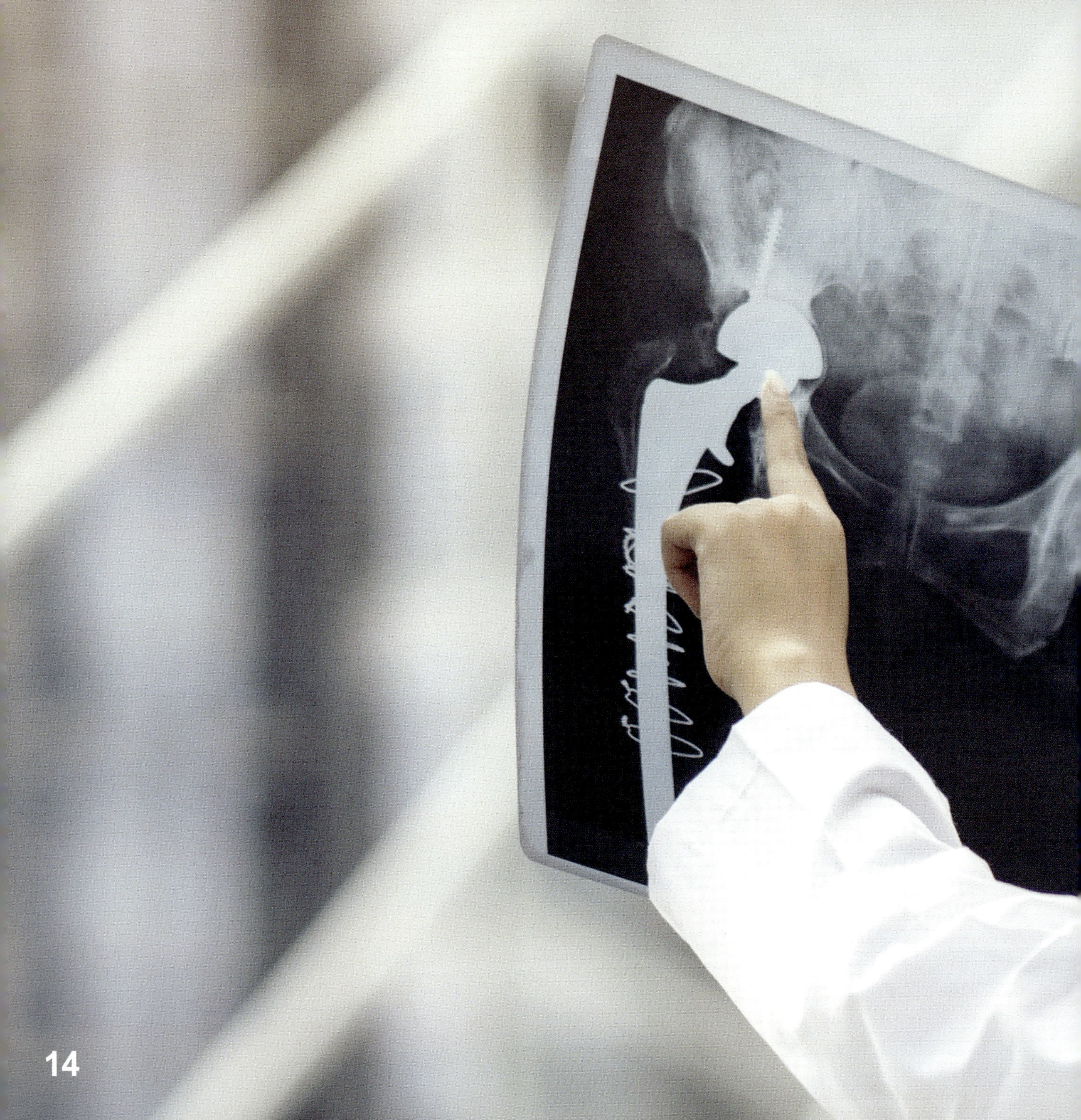

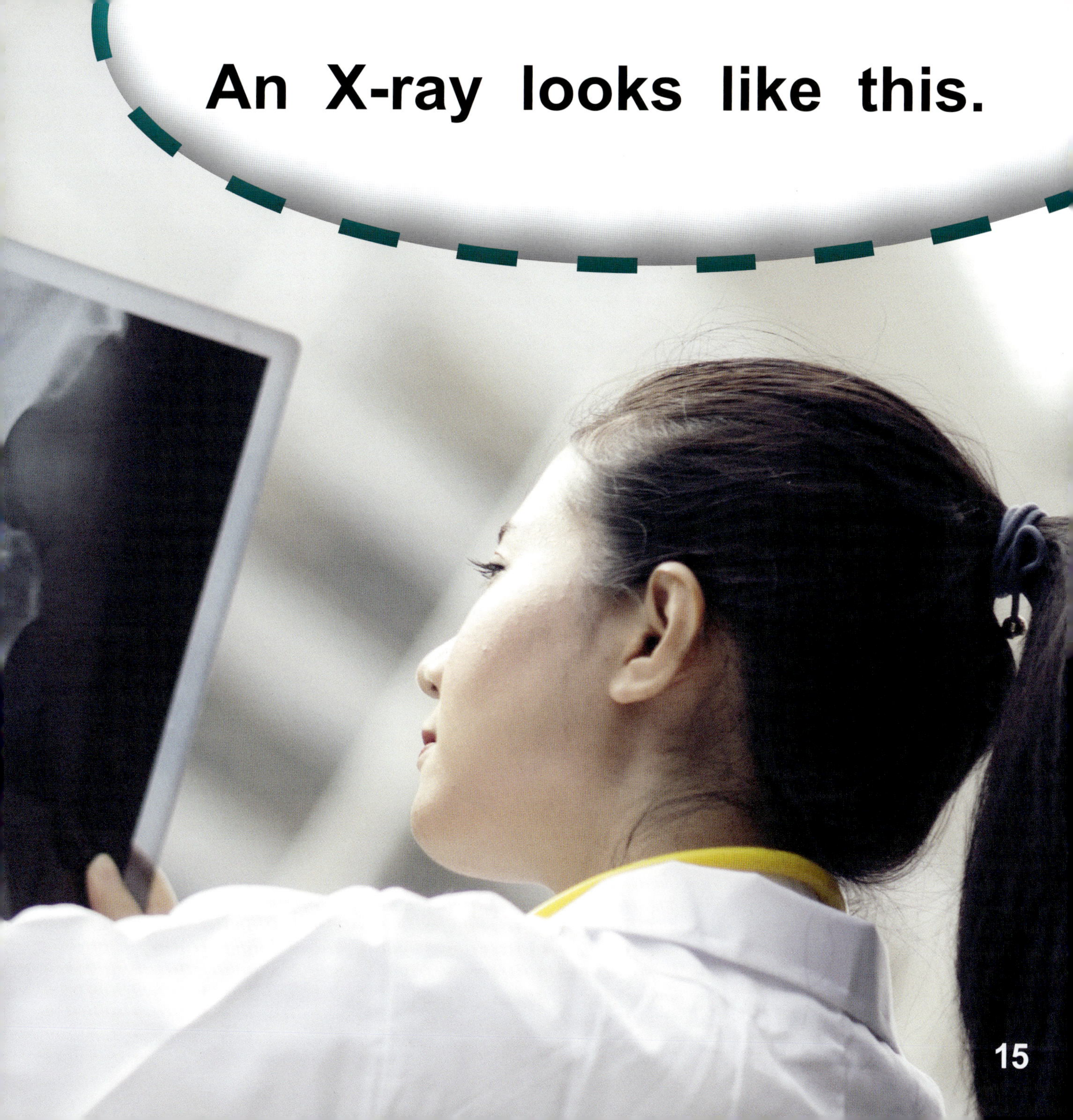

An X-ray looks like this.

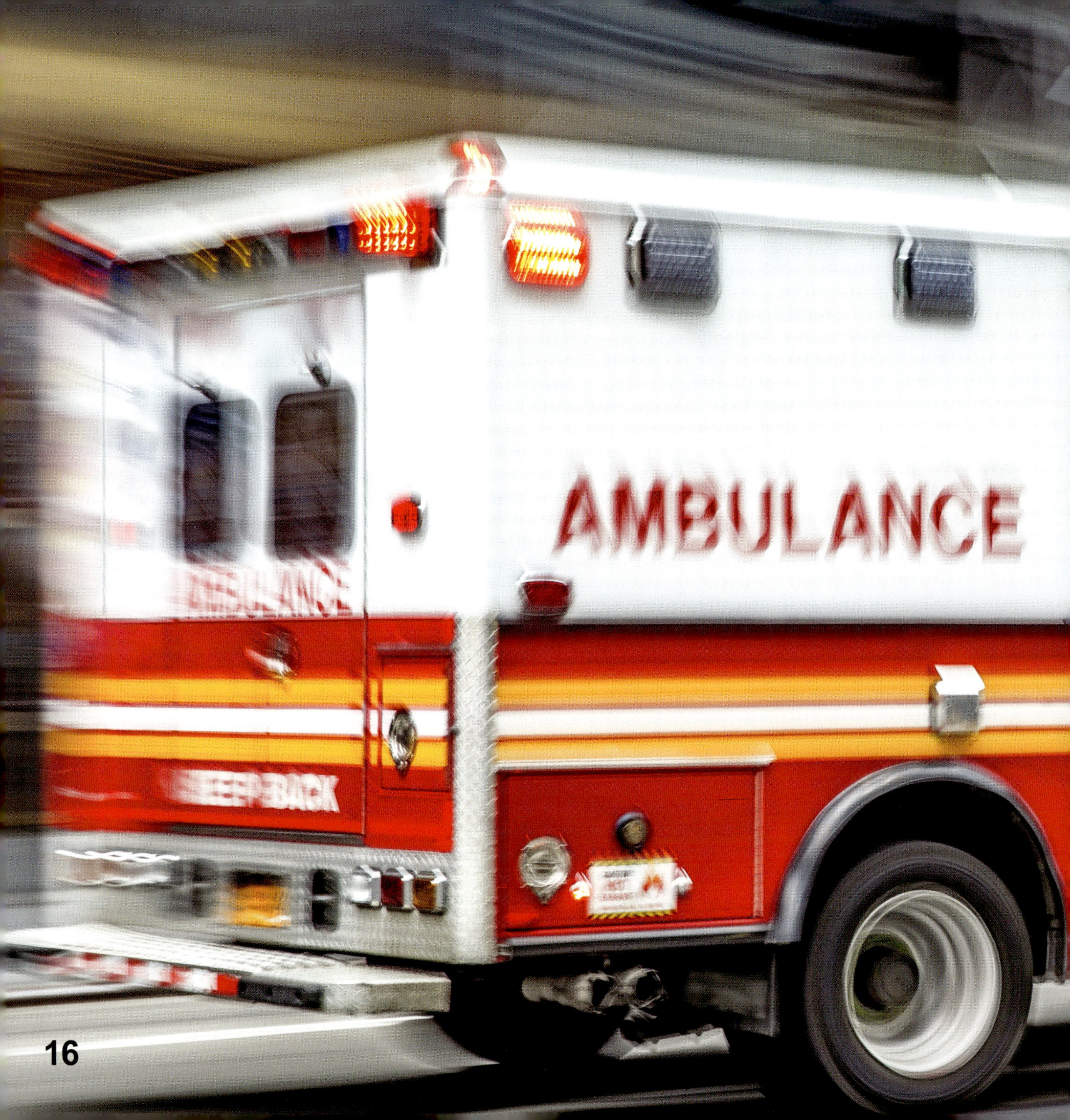
AMBULANCE

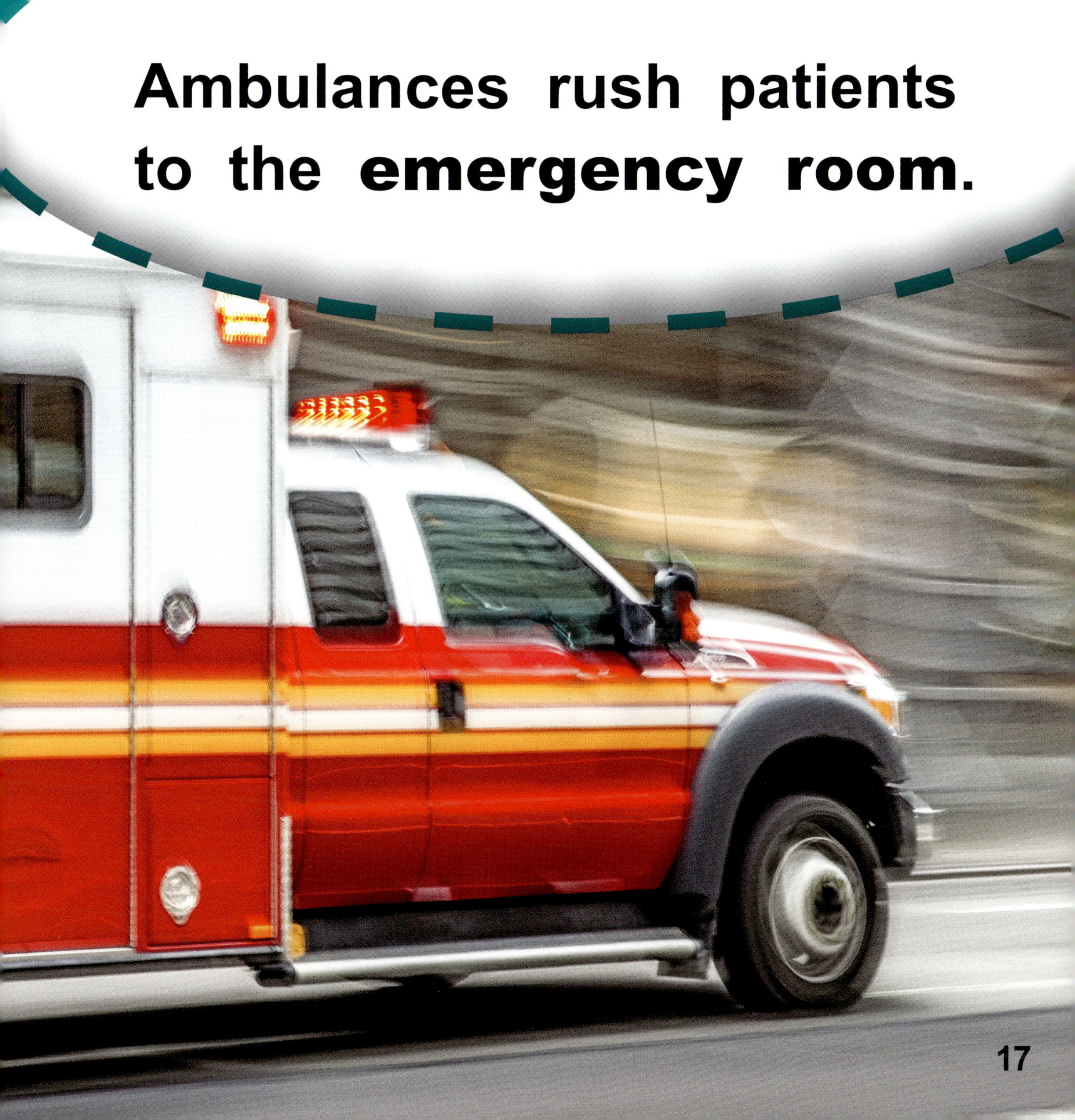

Ambulances rush patients to the **emergency room.**

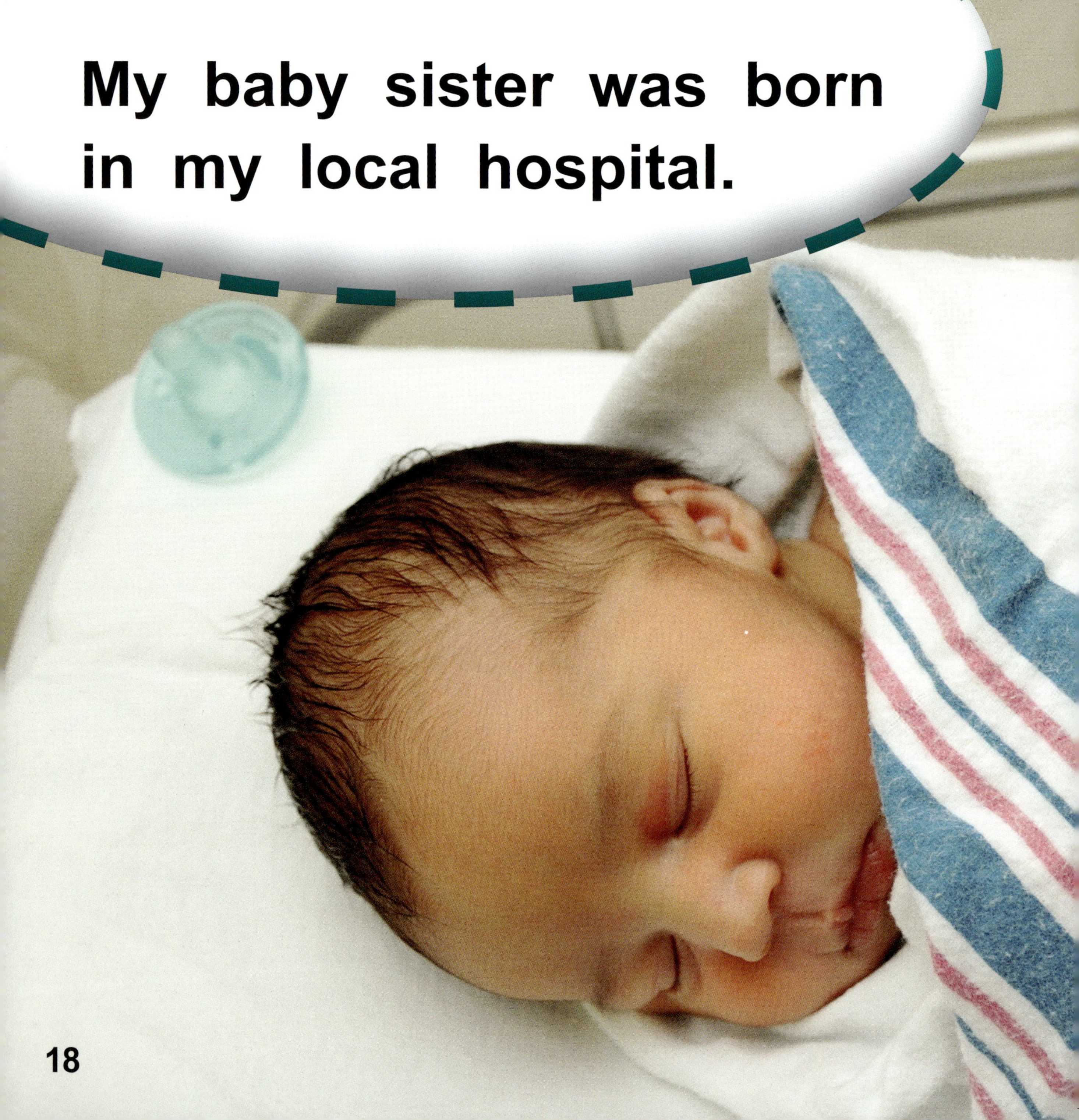

My baby sister was born in my local hospital.

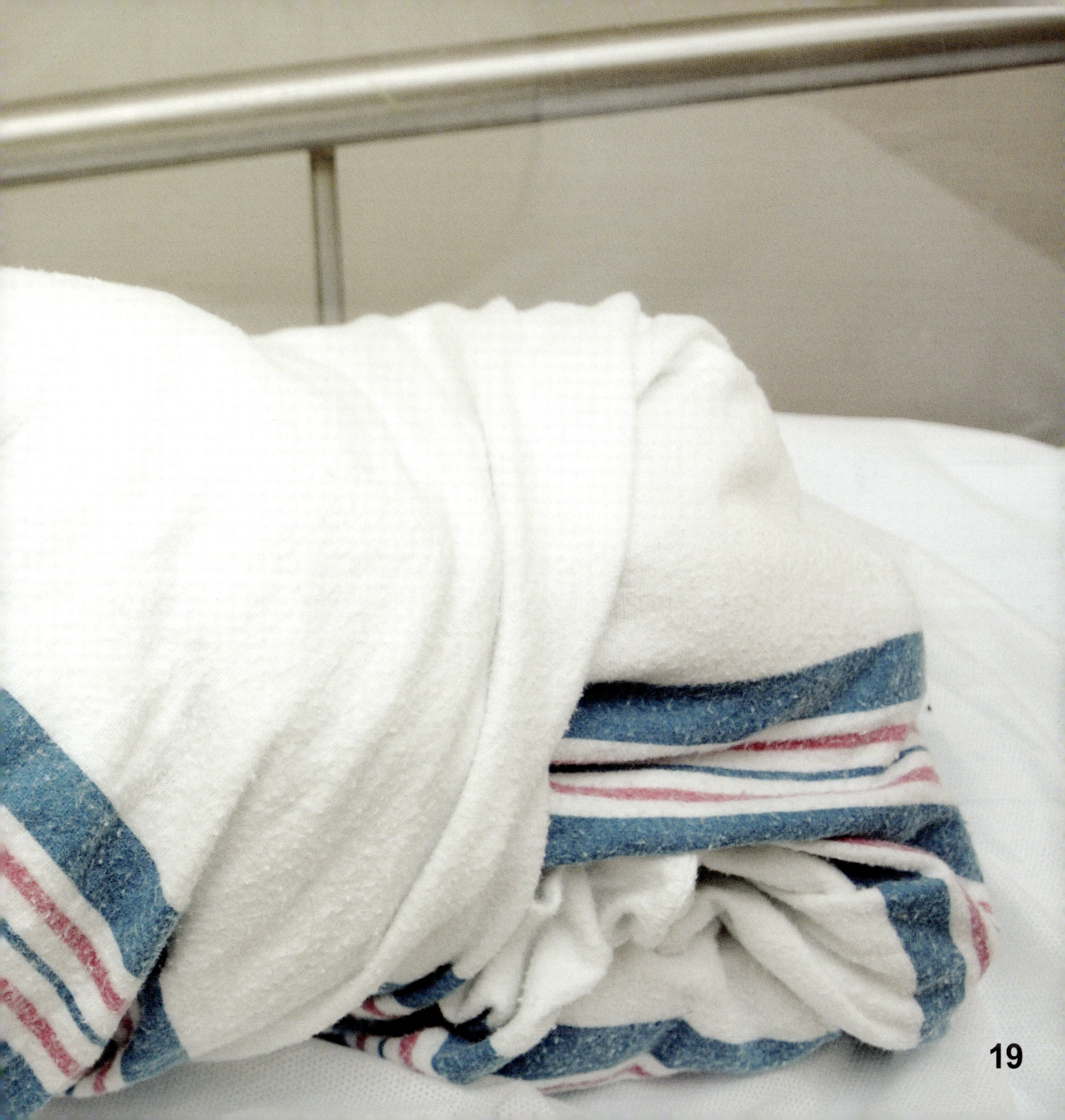

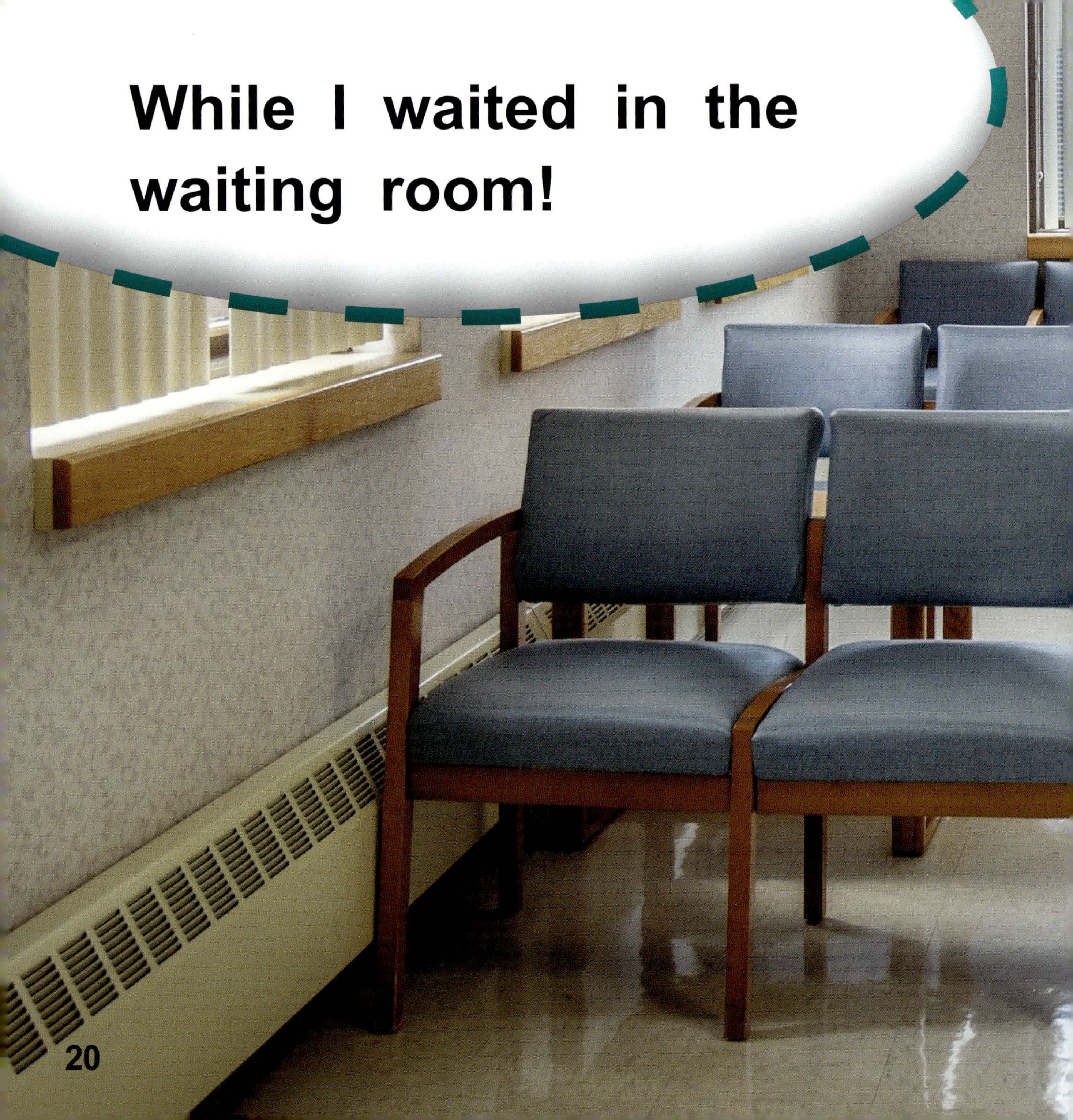

While I waited in the waiting room!

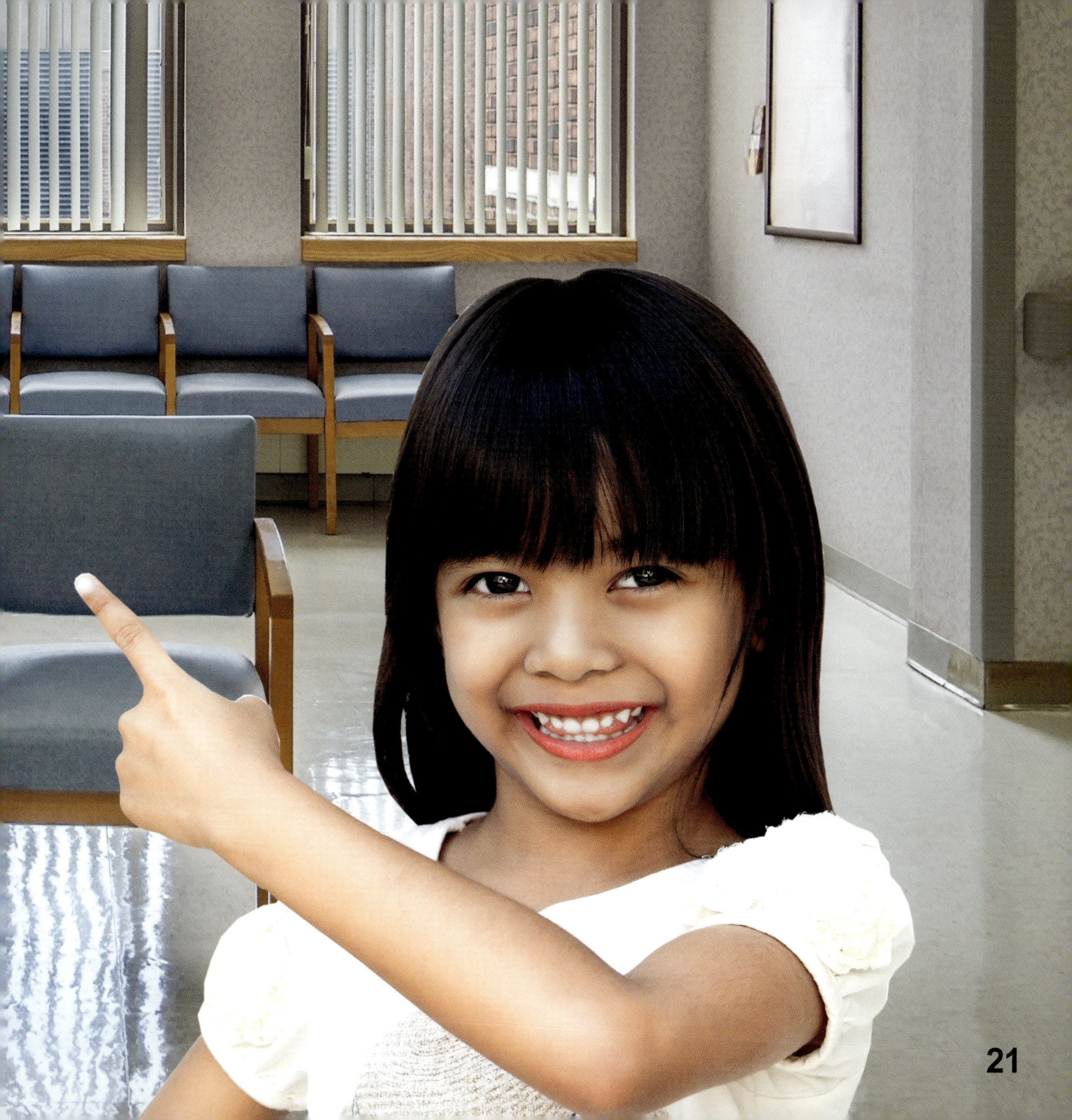

Glossary

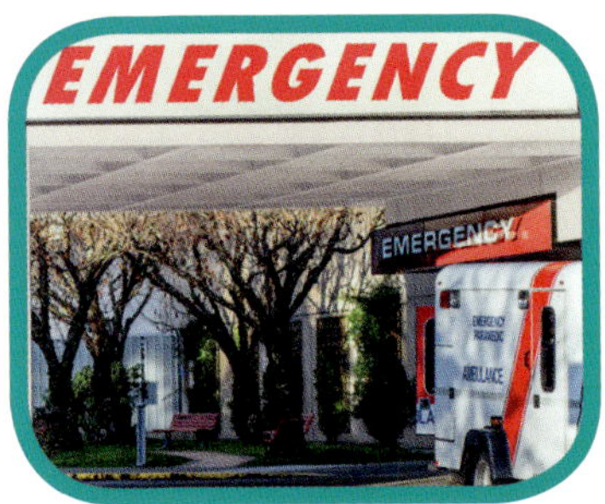

emergency room (i-MUR-jin-see ROOM): An emergency room is where you go if you are badly hurt or sick and need help quickly.

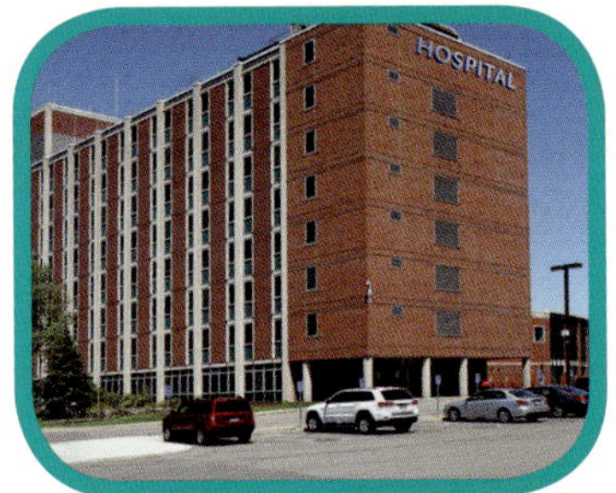

hospital (HOSS-pi-tuhl): A hospital is a place where people go when they are sick or hurt and need special care.

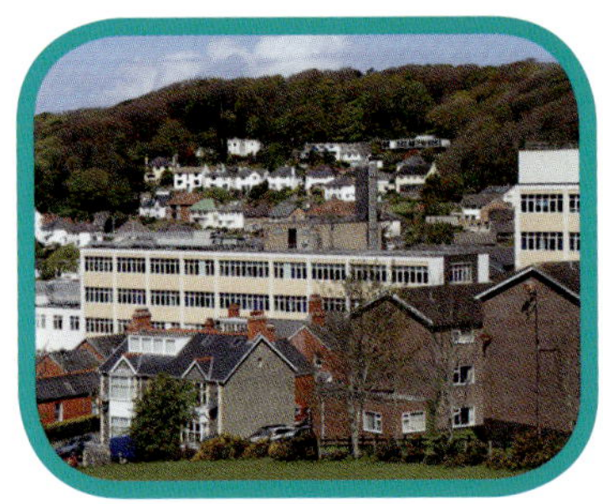

local (LOH-kuhl): Local means close to your house or town.

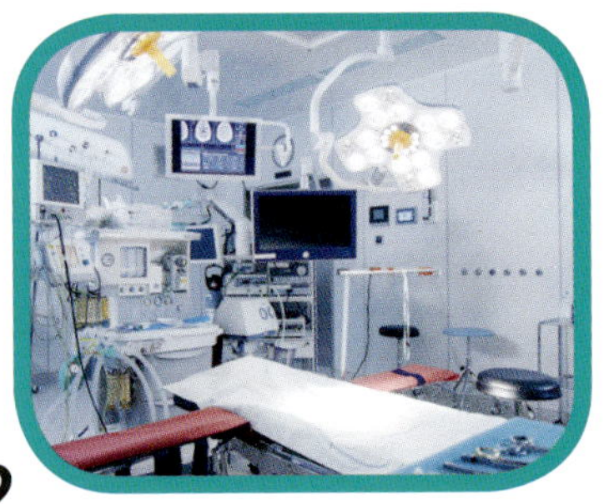

operating room (OP-uh-RATE-ing ROOM): An operating room is where doctors and nurses use special medical tools to repair a patient's body.

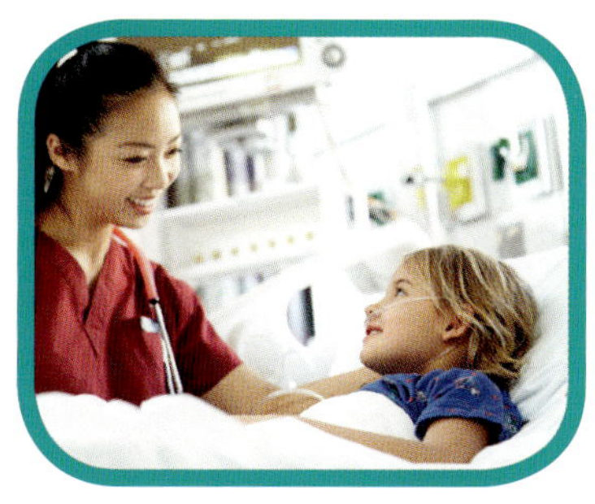

patients (PAY-shuhnts): Patients are sick or hurt people that need a doctor.

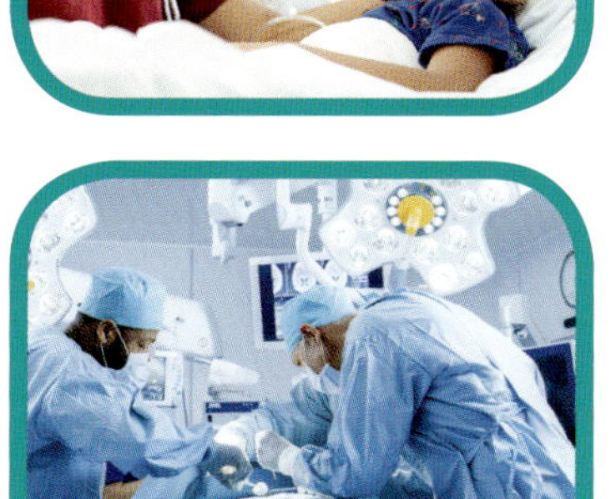

surgery (SUR-jer-ee): Surgery is done by doctors and nurses using special tools to repair a patient's body. The patient is usually in a deep sleep during surgery.

Index

School-to-Home Support for Caregivers and Teachers

Crabtree Seedlings books help children grow by letting them practice reading. Here are a few guiding questions to help the reader with building his or her comprehension skills. Possible answers are included.

Before Reading

- What do I think this book is about? I think this book is about a hospital. It might tell us why hospitals are important.
- What do I want to learn about this topic? I want to learn about the people who work in hospitals.

During Reading

- I wonder why... I wonder why people need X-rays.
- What have I learned so far? I have learned that doctors and nurses work in hospitals.

After Reading

- What details did I learn about this topic? I learned that there are different rooms in a hospital. There are rooms with beds for patients. There is an operating room and an emergency room.
- Read the book again and look for the vocabulary words. I see the word ***surgery*** on page 10 and the word ***emergency room*** on page 17. The other vocabulary words are found on pages 22 and 23.

Library and Archives Canada Cataloging-in-Publication Data

Title: My local hospital / Alan Walker.
Names: Walker, Alan, 1963- author.
Description: Series statement: In my community | "A Crabtree seedlings book". | Includes index.
Identifiers: Canadiana 20200388126 | ISBN 9781427129574 (hardcover) | ISBN 9781427129673 (softcover)
Subjects: LCSH: Hospitals—Juvenile literature.
Classification: LCC RA963.5 .W35 2021 | DDC j362.11—dc23

Library of Congress Cataloging-in-Publication Data

Names: Walker, Alan, 1963- author.
Title: My local hospital / Alan Walker.
Description: New York, NY : Crabtree Publishing Company, [2021] | Series: In my community : a Crabtree seedlings book | Includes index. Identifiers: LCCN 2020050795 | ISBN 9781427129574 (hardcover) | ISBN 9781427129673 (paperback)
Subjects: LCSH: Hospitals--Juvenile literature.
Classification: LCC RA963.5 .W35 2021 | DDC 362.11--dc23
LC record available at https://lccn.loc.gov/2020050795

Crabtree Publishing Company
www.crabtreebooks.com 1-800-387-7650
e-book ISBN 978-1-952398-23-0
Print book version produced jointly with Crabtree Publishing Company NY, USA

Written by Alan Walker
Production coordinator and Prepress technician: Ken Wright
Print coordinator: Katherine Berti

Printed in the U.S.A ./012021/CG20201112

Photo credits: Cover photo © Monkey Business Images, hospital logo © TotemArt, page 2-3 hospital © Spiroview Inc, girl © Patrick Foto; page 4-5 © wavebreakmedia; 6-7 © Monkey Business Images; pages 8-9 and 10011 © Gorodenkoff; page 12-13 © Tyler Olson; page 14-15 © NaruFoto; page 16-17 © blurAZ; page 18-19 © rSnapshotPhotos; page 20-21 © Monkey Business Images, page 22 emergency room © Viktor Birkus, buildings © Wozzie. All photos from Shutterstock.com

Published in Canada
Crabtree Publishing
616 Welland Ave.
St. Catharines, ON
L2M 5V6

Published in the United States
Crabtree Publishing
347 Fifth Ave
Suite 1402-145
New York, NY 10016

Published in the United Kingdom
Crabtree Publishing
Maritime House
Basin Road North, Hove
BN41 1WR

Published in Australia
Crabtree Publishing
Unit 3 – 5
Currumbin Court
Capalaba QLD 4157